Is Your Window Open?

How to eat your way to health and weight loss

Faith Walters

Published by Good News Ministries
220 Sleepy Creek Rd, Macon, Ga 31210
ISBN: 978-1-888081-48-0
Copyright 2019

No portion of this book may be copied or duplicated
without permission

.

Firstly, I am not a doctor or nutritionist, and nothing in this book should be taken as medical advice. I am simply sharing what I have learned. I encourage you to do your own research, and speak with your doctor or nutritionist about any concerns.
I will provide suggested reading material and resources throughout and also at the end.

Secondly, this is a very basic overview. I am not an expert and can not answer questions beyond my scope, especially when it comes to various health conditions. If you want further information and more detailed explanations, please take note of my references and suggested reading material.

I encourage you to do your own research. There is a vast expanse of research, books, documentaries, articles and papers out there. Not all of them will agree with one another, and some might even be contradictory. But don't let that stop you.

The Diet Lie

Frustration. Hunger. Deprivation. Hard Work. Highs. Lows. Commitment. Struggle. Weight. Body Fat. Exercise. Denial. Binging. Depression. Lifestyle. Health. Food. Unfair. Unsustainable.

Those are all words that are often associated with "diet". How many of these words bring happiness when you read them? Not many. Maybe even none. Most of us have been at the point where we have seen food as an enemy that must be defeated. We must deny this or that, we must weigh, count, calculate, reduce, every thing that goes into our mouth. But I have to come to believe, it is ALL a gigantic lie.

When I was a teenager, I started buying low fat, fat free, sugar free (ie: artificially sweetened) and low calorie foods, because I thought that was healthy. I didn't really need to lose weight, but I thought I was making "healthier" food choices. How many of you went this route? How did it work out for you? What has several decades of low fat, low calorie, sugar free and fat free gotten us? One of the largest obese populations in the world. Thank you for those dietary recommendations, geniuses. Uggh.

Fast forward in time and in an effort to lose baby weight after my second child, I embarked on a diet plan that seemed to have lots of merit. You ate 6 times a day, with specific proportions, and a menu of approved foods to choose from. You even got to have one "cheat day" a week, where you could indulge in that favorite treat. And you know what, it worked, sort of. I did lose a little weight, but I didn't FEEL great. I felt pretty ok-ish.

But, at some point, I'm not even sure when, I found myself not following the plan anymore. I mean who has time to eat 6 accurately measured meals a day, with a toddler and a baby? At one point, I was having to purchase their fairly expensive high protein nutrition bars, just to get all the meals in. Ya, no thanks.

Fast forward again to after my third child was born. Uggh. Gained more weight this time than the other two, and it wasn't coming off so easily this time either.

A few years in, and after searching around, and trying a few things here and there, I finally settled on low carb. These were the days of Atkins. Carbs were now my fiercest enemy, that I must defeat at all costs. I bought the shakes, the bars and even the frozen meals, as it was all ready to eat without the carbs. Though it did taste like cardboard. But that's the price you pay. It requires sacrifice. And Yep, sure enough, eventually, I lost all my weight – even to the point of being below my pre-pregnancy weight!

But you know what? I still didn't FEEL good. Passible, functioning, but not GOOD. I stayed on this for quite some time, and kept the weight off. But celebrations, parties, birthdays, holidays and special events happened and I was miserable. Either I had to completely deny that piece of birthday cake and continue to feel no enjoyment from food, or I could "indulge" and by the next day, be completely bloated, gross and 5 pounds heavier. I began to hate it. Plus, I began noticing some health related things that concerned me: bloating, fatigue, inflammation, more frequent headaches, to name a few. At the time, I didn't know why I was having these issues. So I chalked it up to stress and age.

After about a year and half, I slipped back into eating carbs again, and started to gain weight back. Whoops! So I joined a gym and set out on intensive exercise to keep my weight under control. But man, was it hard to get that weight off. It sure seemed to take an extraordinary amount of effort to burn just a tiny amount of calories and drop just a pound or two. I'd look at the little digits on the elliptical or treadmill and think

"That's it? That's all the calories I've burned? You've got to be kidding me!"

And the over exertion and overheating triggered horrible migraines, and the extra exercise made me so hungry, I was eating more than ever! Needless to say, this was not working well for me either.

By this time I was really struggling with inflammation, chronic fasciitis, chronic fatigue, chronic migraines, swollen, achy feet and legs, and just feeling bad most of the time. Every so often I would have a good, pain free, moderate energy day, and I just would wish it could last, but it never did. I began to search out all kinds of supplements, vitamins and natural remedies. And eventually after much trial and error and much money spent, I did find some that really helped. They did make me feel better, though still not great, but they kept me functioning. However, I knew that couldn't be the total answer. I wanted to feel not just ok, or even good. I wanted to feel great.

Eventually I learned about your gut balance and its effect on your whole health. It actually started with my daughter, who was struggling with stomach and digestive issues, that her pediatrician couldn't help. Prescription anti-acid and anti-reflux meds was their answer, but they didn't help. And my thought was that it is just not normal or right to have a little girl on meds like that. We needed to heal the root problem, not just try and control the symptoms with medication. So I began to search for answers.

While this was happening, I began having awful coughing fits, that lasted for weeks and months at a time. The doctor gave me mucinex, allergy pills and nasal spray. They did nothing. I went back and they just suggested a different brand of allergy medicine. But that didn't change anything either.

So I decided to see an allergist, to see if I could pin point what was causing this and if there was perhaps a food allergy triggering it. Well, $1000 later, I had NO allergies! A little perplexed, the allergist finally had a possible diagnosis. Silent Reflux. It's like acid relfux, except you don't get the burning sensation in your chest (thus the silent), and your stomach acids shoot all the way up into your sinuses, then drip back down, causing the awful coughing fits. Awesome.

I was sent home with a reflux prescription. Uggh. More medicine? I, like my daughter, wanted to be better, not just try to control symptoms with a lifetime of medication. Instead, because I was learning a little about the gut bacteria, and put two and two together that my reflux was coming from my stomach, I decided to try to attack this as naturally as possible. Thanks to a suggestion from a friend, I started taking apple cider vinegar and occasionally baking soda in water instead. Worked like a charm.

Back to my daughter. I began to realize her issue was gut balance related too. We spent the next few months working on bringing our gut back into balance. We started with some probiotics from our local health food store, and daily doses of apple cider vinegar. I then took a class and learned to make kombucha and that has been a staple in our house ever since. Both my daughter and I have had great results. Why is this important you wonder? It's very important. I will tie in gut health later in the book, in "Listen to your Gut".

My gut was healing, but my weight was still an issue. By now I was in my 40's and it seemed like no matter what I did, I was just gaining little by little each year. Maybe just 5 lbs here, 5 lbs there, but it was like it had a mind of its own and it was starting to add up. And I just didn't know what to do anymore. I wanted to give up. So I resigned myself to just perpetually be 20-30lbs overweight.

So, let's get back to the dirty word "diet". We've seen and heard it all: CICO (calories in, calories out), Low Fat, Low Calorie, High Fat, Low Carb, No Carb, High Protein, Vegetarian, Keto, Paleo, Vegan,

Carnivore, Weight Watchers, Jenny Craig, Atkins, the list goes on and on and on. And on. They can't all be right. Or can they? Why does ____ work for so and so, but didn't work for you? Most likely people will say it's because you didn't try hard enough, or didn't commit long enough. They want you to know their diet WORKS, you just aren't doing it right. You have failed. Shame on you. But that is likely untrue. More often than not, the "diet" fails us, not the other way around.

With so many diets, and so much contradicting information, something is amiss. If you have stumbled into a diet that works for you – meaning not just that you are at healthy weight, but you are HAPPY, you are HEALHTY and your body is physically happy, mentally happy, you are at peace and rest, you sleep well, have good energy, and you are not controlled by food (whether eating too much, or obsessed with counting points, carbs, calories, macros, ounces, grams etc.) then you are very fortunate. It's much harder for most of us. I am a living testimony that just because you aren't severely overweight, doesn't mean you are healthy.

The Three Biggest Lies

1. CICO: Calories in, Calories out: Or the "Eat less, Move more" phenomenon. You need to eat less calories to lose weight. NOT! A calorie is a measurement of the rate at which something burns, or energy is expended. But your body has no idea what calories are. It couldn't care less what amount of calories a food item has. It doesn't compute. Weight is not regulated by calories, it is regulated by hormones. Read that again. Hormones are what tell your body to store fat, or release fat, not calories. It is actually not dependent on how many calories you eat or restrict. Your body will adjust to your calorie intake through your signals sent by hormones.

If you restrict calories, you may lose some weight initially, but your body will adjust its energy expenditure to match the intake, lowering your metabolism. If your body sees that over time it is consistently receiving less energy in, it will adjust the energy you put out so as not to cause a deficit. That is why anyone who does a restrictive calorie diet, always puts the weight back on, and finds it even harder to get off the next time. We will talk about this more in depth in the next chapter.

2. The Food Pyramid and Dietary Recommendations. For the most part, people tend to follow these. So why is our population filled with obesity, diabetes, heart disease, auto-immune disorders, gastro and metabolic disorders? You can only assume these recommendations can't possibly be valid. Plus, they change every few years! Eggs are bad, then eggs were good but only the whites, now eggs with yolk are good. Dairy is bad, dairy is good.

Fats are bad, now fats are good again. It'll make your head spin.

3. If you just exercise more, you will lose weight. This ties into the "Eat less, Move more" theory. Though exercise is very good for your body and heart, and helps to tone and strengthen muscle, it is not actually an efficient way to lose weight. Out of our Total Energy (or calorie) Expenditure, only about 5% is consumed by physical activity. Total Energy Expenditure overwhelmingly (about 95%) comes from your Basal Metabolic Rate: which takes care of tasks such as breathing, maintaining body temperature, pumping the heart, brain function, vital organ function, liver and kidney function etc. We treat exercise like its equal partners with food when it comes to weight. But it simply isn't. It plays a much smaller role. And furthermore, decreased calorie intake, can reduce your basal metabolic rate by up to 40%, while increased calorie intake can increase it by as much as 50%.

That is quite a bit more effective than an hour on a treadmill.

We were never designed or created to "diet". It's just not compatible. It's not how our bodies work. Look around in your local Walmart, mall, or any public place and it is very evident. We are the most health and diet conscience we've ever been, more technologically and medically advanced than we've ever been, yet, we are the sickest and fattest we've ever been! Seventy percent, of Americans are on at least one prescription drug, Another study puts the numbers at 3 out of 5. One in five kids ages 12-19 are obese. And almost 40% of adults over 20 are obese. There is something very wrong with this picture. We need real answers.

I could write another whole book on the problems with disease and health/healthcare. But many have already done that. If you want to dive deeper into that area, then I suggest starting with a documentary called "The Business of Disease. It is available on Amazon, and is free to Prime members. There are plenty of books and articles on the problems with the health industry. So we won't concentrate on that aspect in this book. We are going to focus on food health.

Ready Set Weight

Look at the course of obesity and obesity related diseases over the decades. It is obvious to anyone the trend has significantly increased as years have gone by. Before the 1950's and 1960's, most of the population ate 3 meals a day: breakfast, lunch and dinner, and less during the times of the Great Depression. There was almost no processed food, except for maybe bleached white flour and refined white sugar, which was often used more sparingly. And obesity was much more rare. And 150 years ago it was almost unheard of.

Now in more recent years we've been told we must eat 5-6 times a day for energy and to boost metabolism. Highly processed, nutrient lacking food is often upwards of 80% of typical American diets. And obesity has doubled since the 1980's. The whole rigamarole of low fat, fat free, low calorie and zero calorie food and drinks has been one of our greatest detriments to health and weight. All of these foods are highly processed to remove the calories and fats, and are replaced with chemicals made in a lab to make them palatable. Often times additives like MSG are added to cause you to crave these foods. And thanks to all this, here we are, with the highest obesity rates and highest metabolic disorder rates in history. It's obviously not about the fat or calories. So something is not right.

Studies have been done to understand what that could be. And guess what? Eating more often, will cause you to gain more, regardless of calories. What a notion! It doesn't matter if you eat or drink a low or even zero calorie item. It has been shown that diet sodas lead to weight gain just as much as regular soda, sometimes even more so.

Like I said before, your body does not compute calories. Calories are not equal. The calories in a tablespoon of olive oil, are not equal to the same amount of calories in sugar. Your body metabolizes them differently. So we can not reliably measure food by calories, when the metabolic response is different to different foods. And we know that weight is not controlled by calories, but .by hormones: insulin, cortisol, ghrelin and leptin among others. And the main driving factor of them all is insulin.

Scientists have learned that every time you eat, there is a glucose response in your body that causes a spike in insulin. When this happens frequently, and insulin stays high for long periods of time, the insulin signals your body to store what you eat and drink. Your body stores it in two ways – glycogen and fat.

The body stores glycogen first, as it

is easily accessible to be turned back into energy. But when glycogen stores get full, the body then stores fat, which is more of a long term storage and harder to access. When this happens, excessive glycogen and fat stores lead to fatty liver disease, obesity, heart problems, diabetes and an array of metabolic disorders.

So the more often we eat, and spike our insulin, the more our bodies store fat. And the more our insulin levels stay raised, the more it effects our other hormones. After time, we become insulin resistant and also become leptin resistant.

Leptin is the hormone that sends us our signal that we are full and need to stop eating. We end up over eating, because our leptin resistance stops us from knowing when to stop, and we just keep feeling hungry. This is actually a result of obesity (or insulin resistance), not the cause. Unless our insulin lowers, and remains so for a significant period of time, our bodies will not burn through our stored glycogen. And if we can't burn through our stored glycogen, we can't access our stored fat.

Another factor in weight gain is cortisol. I am not going to talk much about cortisol, except to say that cortisol is released due to stress. When we experience stress, cortisol signals our bodies to release glucose into our blood. This is meant to give us a surge of extra energy, in a fight or flight type situation. After a time, it subsides. Logic tells us that this would cause a burning of glycogen, which contributes to weight loss, and this is true. But when we have a constant release of cortisol due to our over stressed lifestyles, it actually works against insulin, as insulin is disrupted and can't regulate glucose properly, thus causing weight gain. It is VERY important to find ways to reduce stress in your life. It is true that too much stress for too long, will disrupt your insulin and cause weight gain.

An additional interesting aspect of this is that we all have an internal set weight point that our bodies will ALWAYS return to. Dr. Jason Fung uses a great analogy of a thermostat. The thermostat in our home, will constantly adjust the temperature, to maintain the set point. No matter the temperature outside, or what happens inside, it will always work to keep the temperature at the set point. Through our lifestyle and diet habits, many of us have inadvertently entered our weight set point way too high, ironically, usually from dieting and restricting calories.

But when we try to "diet" our way back down, our bodies are fighting us, working to keep us at the set point that is currently entered. That is a big reason why we gain, we lose, and we gain it right back again. The only way to fix that, it to reset that weight set point.

There is still yet another very important function in our bodies, that is the key to health, weight and healing, that is greatly affected by our insulin levels. It's called autophagy.

Autophagy is our body's natural recycling: it is the process in which old, damaged, unnecessary and dysfunctional cells are disassembled and degraded to make way for new, clean healthy cells. It the perfect rebuilding machine. Illness and disease are caused by damaged and unhealthy cells in our bodies.

If we can help our body become more efficient at replacing these cells with new healthy cells, then we will be much more healthy over all. And when we are constantly digesting and causing insulin spikes, it greatly reduces this process. So not only are we telling our bodies to store fat and glucose, through constant insulin raising, we are also inhibiting one of our most vital natural processes. Lowering insulin levels not only promotes autophagy, but increases it. This is where significant healing of the body and brain takes place. One of my favorite concise explantions of autophagy can be found at www. DietDoctor.com/renew-body-fasting-autophagy

A Nobel Prize winning study by Yoshinori Ohsumi,
https://www.nobelprize.org/nobel_prizes/medicine/laureates/2016.html
noted that disrupted and disturbed autophagy was linked to Parkinson's, type 2 diabetes, and cancer, among other diseases; and mutations in autophagy are linked to genetic diseases.

But there is good news: an effective and simple way to balance our hormones, and promote both autophagy and weight loss is our for the taking. It's all in the timing.

Timing is Everything

For tens of thousands of years, our ancestors did not sit down to their three, (or 6) meals a day. They didn't go to their fridge or their nearest drive thru every time they were bored or wanted a little snack. They hunted, gathered, worked, and sowed and reaped, and then ate. And they definitely had no concept of what a calorie was. Or carbs. Or points. Or even macro or micro nutrients. And when they ate, they usually ate quite a bit.

Think back over history, there was a lot of feasting. There were many occasions for feasting: religious feasts, harvest feasts, wedding feasts, holiday feasts – they sure like to feast! But there wasn't an obesity epidemic. Why? It was balanced with times of not eating. Our ancestors did not feast continually, or even eat throughout the day. They ate periodically, and almost never regularly.

Did you know the average American today eats up to 50 times a week? FIFTY! Think about that. FIFTY. When our body is that busy trying desperately to regulate insulin and digest all this food, it has little time to do anything else. You will never be able to achieve efficient autophagy, lose weight and keep it off, or reset the weight set point with insulin continually high.

The Window

Just like opening a window in our house to let the fresh air in, opening up a window for eating, allows us let the nourishment in, appropriately. But the thing about the window, whether in our house or with our food, is after a period of time, we close it again. We have periods of open windows and closed windows.

When your window is closed, in the realm of food, you are in what's called a fasting state. We are in a fasting state every night while we sleep. Going through periods of fasting, allows your body to take a break and focus on other vital processes, like autophagy and proper hormone regulation. It allows our bodies to enter into metabolic rest, which lowers our glucose levels, normalizing insulin and other hormones like gherlin (which sends the hunger signal), leptin (which tells us when to stop eating), and HGH (promotes lean muscle mass).

If these extremely important hormones are out of balance, we will never succeed and never be able to reset the weight set point. And extending this period of fasting beyond our sleep, is extremely beneficial.

Now don't be scared by the word fasting. And no, research shows that your body does not enter into "starvation mode" and tank your metabolism or burn up all your muscle for energy. That's what extreme calorie reduction does. Actually, with fasting, the opposite has been proven to be true.

There was a study that was done on the contestants of The Biggest Loser: If you aren't familiar with the tv show, it is a contest with very obese people who were put on a severe calorie restricted diet with intense exercise, and they saw who could lose the most weight by the end. And boy! Do they lose a lot of weight! BUT it was discovered that their basal metabolic rate (metabolism) plummeted, and remained so.... more than 6 years later. No wonder almost all of them gained their weight back. Their bodies adapted to lower calorie intake, by compensating with lower calorie output, lowering their metabolism.
See: idmprogram.com/biggest-loser-diet-explained/

On the flip side, it has been shown

that by fasting, your metabolism INCREASES. See: https://www.ncbi.nlm.nih.gov/pubmed/1083 7292

Through fasting, hormones such as insulin, gherlin, leptin and HGH are properly regulated and the body begins to heal itself much more efficiently. And increased HGH actually helps build lean muscle, not the other way around. You tap into those glycogen stores for energy, and then into the fat stores and your body boosts your metabolism, to keep up with the demand. Everything we thought we knew, was wrong.

We've already discussed what lowering your glucose and regulating insulin does, but another interesting factor comes with the proper regulation of gherlin and leptin – remember, those are the hunger and full hormones. When those are properly working, we will not overeat. And fasting gets those back into balance. After a period of fasting, when you've adapted, (which takes a different amount of time for different people) you achieve a state called "appetite correction", which is when those hormones are balanced again. When they are balanced, and you are not in the range of being insulin or leptin resistant, you can trust your body to tell you when you've had enough to eat. Over eating will not be a problem, because your hormones will be balanced, and your signals will be clear and uninterrupted.

For further study on this, read *AC: The Power of Appetite Correction* by Dr. Bert Herring. For an in depth look on all of what I have been talking about, and more, Also, read *The Obesity Code* by Jason Fung, MD.

I want to recommend reading www.idmprogram.com/fix-broken-metabolim/. And watching a great video by Dr. Jason Fung, that really explains all of this much better than I can. It can be found on youtube by searching "Therapeutic Fasting – Solving the Two-Compartment Problem", or by entering this link: https://youtu.be/tluj-oMN-Fk.

Fasting is also incredibly beneficial for the brain and for neurodegenerative disorders such as Alzheimer's and Parkinson's. So many studies are being done on this. It has been shown that fasting improves cognitive function, increases neuropathic factors, neurogenesis, and increases stress resistance. For further study on this, start with watch a youtube video TEDx called "Why fasting bolsters brain power: Mark Mattson" and then go from there.

How and When

The How: If you do any searching online about fasting, you will find a wide array of opinions and regimens. There are many approaches and I will talk about some of them. However, whatever regimen you go for, there is ONE point in particular that I want to stress. And that is what is known as "**clean fasting**".

We have learned that what we eat and drink causes an insulin response, and the key to all of this it to limit that. So it is crucial that you fast cleanly. Otherwise, it's not even fasting. Drinking diet sodas, juice, flavored water, bulletproof or flavored coffee, herbal teas etc. WILL cause a spike in insulin. It doesn't matter if its "sugar free", "natural flavor" or "zero calorie". Our taste receptors will still tell our insulin that we are eating. If you do some research, you will find some fasters allow these things, but I challenge you clean fast for 30 days and you will discover the undeniable difference for yourself.

So during the fast, it is only acceptable to drink plain water, plain sparkling water, black unflavored coffee (not flavored coffee beans), plain black tea or plain green tea (watch out for teas in particular, as they can have things like citrus, mint, added flavor, or hidden sweeteners, so check the ingredients label. Also matcha is not an acceptable green tea while fasting as you are ingesting leaves).

And sorry, but no, you can not add collagen or MCT oil to your coffee, or fruit or herbs to your tea or water. You can do that when its your eating window. Note: in the fasting community, your time when you are eating is generally referred to as your "window". It is also recommended to not chew gum or mints while fasting, as that activates insulin as well. A small amount of peppermint oil or WOW drops can be used sparingly for bad breath.

There are a few items that are considered in the "grey area", and that is because they cause issues for some people, and not for others. It is recommended to clean fast for at least 4-6 weeks, so you know how that feels, before attempting to add any of the grey area items. These items include:

Cinnamon
Lemon or lime wedge in water
Apple Cider Vinegar
Peppermint essential oil
Other teas

If, after you are adapted to clean fasting, you decide to add one of these items during your fast, and become hungry, shaky or fasting becomes difficult, you know this item is not ok during your fast.

Clean fasting is the only rule I am going to give you regarding fasting. In fact, it is the only rule I'm going to give you period. More on that later. So that's it for the "how". Now on to "when". When do you open your "window" to receive in all the nutrients that fuel our body and brains?

There are many approaches to when you should fast and when you should open your window, and for how long. This part will be up to you and what works with your body, lifestyle and schedule. There are two main fasting strategies: Intermittent fasting and Extended fasting. A great short introductory video on fasting can be found on youtube by searching "What is Intermittent Fasting" on Diet Dcotor's channel. Or by entering http://youtu.be/VlhhrYjVhOk

Intermittent Fasting

Intermittent fasting (IF) is exactly what it sounds like. You fast intermittently. Or eat intermittently. However you want to look at it. It is also sometimes referred to as Time Restricted Eating (Tre). It's shorter fasts on a daily/weekly basis, and is a great place to begin. For the daily basis (TRe), you fast for a certain number of hours per day, and eat for a certain number of hours per day. The hours are always consecutive. In many blogs and posts online you will see ratios like 16:8 or 18:6. These refer to the hours fasting and the hours feasting, (feasting being a favorite term of many fasters in place of eating). 16 being the hours fasted, and 8 being the window open for eating.

Most people start with the 16:8 ratio. If you are reasonably healthy, have moderate portion control and don't eat 6 times a day or are already used to skipping a meal, this will be fairly easy. It is basically either skipping breakfast, or skipping dinner. However, if you struggle with constant eating, and this proves to be too difficult, it is perfectly fine to start with a lower fasting ratio, such as 14:10 o r even 12:12 and gradually work your way up. But for true benefit, you need to get to at least 16:8. So if you need to start low, add 30 min every few days, or an hour a week, or whatever you can handle to gradually increase your time.

You can also begin by first cutting out snacks and eating only three meals a day. Then cut out one of the meals. If you find it particularly difficult, some people start with a "fat fast". It is designed for people who are used to eating a large amount of carbohydrates and have a hard time adapting to fasting. IF you feel like you may need to start with this, you can read about the protocol on www.idmprogram.com/what-is-fat-fasting-and-when-you-should-do-it/

However you start, you will need about 2-4 weeks period to initially adapt and strengthen that fasting muscle. After all, we are used to eating all the time, especially when that afternoon slump or the "hanger" sets in. We reach for that quick energy, that is often something sweet, or carby that gives us an instant insulin spike. But we all know what happens just a short time later – that dreaded crash. Then we are back for more food and to another quick insulin spike. And so the cycle continues. We never have true sustainable energy that way. It can even happen with "healthy food". We are constantly receiving energy from the food we eat, instead of tapping into all the wonderful and sustainable energy we have just sitting in our system.

Once you find that 16:8 is easy, doable and even enjoyable, you can begin to experiment with different ratios. Not everyone can lose all the weight they need with 16:8, or they hit a plateau and need an extra push. Many people increase to 18:6, 19:5, 20:4 etc. When and if you get into the ranges of 19:5 or greater, you are entering into an eating style known as "OMAD" or one meal a day. Don't let that scare you, It does NOT mean one plate a day. Author Gin Stephens defines OMAD as eating up to three times (think like going out for a meal – snack/appetizer, meal and dessert, eaten within a 5 hour period or less). And YES! You CAN have dessert!

Now this may sound scary or restrictive. But it's not. Trust me. If its too much to consider right now, and sounds impossible, just remember, this is not where most people would start, and is not even required to see the benefits of fasting. Its a choice some people make, and many even naturally gravitate to over time. So go slow if you need to. This is not a race, its a journey. You listen to your body and do what you can, when you can.

I mentioned before about something called "appetite correction". This plays a major role in fasting. This will happen to anyone who is clean fasting for a length of time. It usually doesn't happen to those who fast with juice, flavored water, creamed or sweetened coffee etc. because they are still causing frequent insulin spikes. "Dirty fasting" as its frequently called (though it's not actually fasting) just makes you stay hungry during the fast, making it more difficult to stick with it. This is why some people give up because they are always hungry and don't see the weight loss they hoped for. That is just another reason the clean part of fasting is so important.

Appetite correction happens at different times for different people, depending on how long you fast and how much glycogen stores you have to burn through. When you initially begin fasting, your body accesses those glycogen stores first, and your hormones Ghrelin and Leptin (the hunger and satiety hormones) are on a certain cycle that they are used to.

The first few days or so, you may feel it: maybe slight headache, dizziness, mental fog, acid reflux, those dreaded cravings, even some tiredness are a few side effects. Your body will want you to reach for that instant insulin rush, because that's what it's used to. But as your body recognizes it's not going to get that, it will tap into those glycogen stores. This is when people start to feel better. Energy will start to increase and you won't feel quite as "hungry". But you may have to fight through pretend hunger – like emotional or boredom eating. But you will quickly recognize the difference between true hunger, and eating out of habit, emotions or boredom. And hunger (Ghrelin) always comes in waves, and always subsides again. Anyone who has ever worked through lunch, because you are too busy to stop and eat, knows that after a while, the hunger subsides. So, no you won't just keep increasing in hunger until you die!

Many common initial side effects of fasting can include, headache, dizziness, muscle cramps, diarrhea, constipation, mental fog, lethargy, insomnia, bad breath etc. I know, I know, sounds delightful. But keep in mind they are very temporary. And often can be a sign your electrolytes are out of balance. In this case, supplement with Pink Himalayan or pure Sea salts and magnesium citrate (great for constipation), glycinate, chloride or malate. Magnesium oxide is poorly absorbed in the body, so avoid this kind. Potassium is not generally recommended to supplement, because if your salt and magnesium are good, your potassium will be stable. However, if potassium is needed in the case of an extended fast, it is recommended to **never** exceed 500-1000mg per day, unless prescribed by your doctor. And if you do need potassium, it is best to get it in food form. I will include a simple chart at the end of the chapter to help you with electrolytes.

In a fasted state, you can use coarse salt under your tongue, left to dissolve, or add to coffee or warm water. It is suggested to begin with ¼ tsp of salt and increase as necessary. I add ¼ tsp of sea salt and pink Himalayan salt mixture to my coffee every morning (it cuts the bitterness too!). Many people prefer a topical magnesium oil, instead of an oral supplement for faster absorption and you don't have to worry if it will disrupt an empty stomach.

If that doesn't help or you get to the point of being nauseas, faint feeling, or ill, you might be trying to do too much too soon. If at any point you get sick, always stop. End the fast, eat, then scale back your ratio for a few days, and then try to gradually increase, maybe by just 15 minutes each day if that's what you can do. You will feel waves of hunger, but they pass, usually in 15-30 minutes. Drink some water and distract yourself with something. Many people find that sparkling water (remember to keep it plain!) and green tea help stave off hunger. Take note of the time, and stick to that time for the next day. Then increase that time frame by an hour, or even just 15-30 minutes if an hour is too much, and see what you can do.

Stay hydrated with water, but don't feel you have to drink gallons and gallons. You can actually flush out your electrolytes and minerals by drinking too much, which will lead to lightheadedness and headaches. I drink as I am thirsty. I average 1-3 refills of my 32 oz tumbler per day. Remember during activity or in summer heat, you will need more water than at other times.

When you start reaching the bottom of your glycogen stores (which could be anywhere from 2 weeks – 2 months or more, depending on how much glycogen you have stored up and how long and often you fast), you may suddenly feel more tired or cranky again. This usually does not last long, if you persist. You now have a choice, either allow your body to enter ketosis and tap into that stored fat, or binge and eat your way to increased insulin spikes again.

Ketosis is the the process in which your body's energy comes from ketones in the blood, that are produced by your body metabolizing fat. Once you tap into those fat stores, everything changes.

Appetite correction and adaptation to burning fat for incredibly sustainable energy kicks in. You will notice you aren't hungry when your not supposed to be and your portion control will fully be regulated by your body via your now properly working leptin hormone. Your energy will sustain you all day, with no slumps or crashes, your mind will be focused and clear, and you will see differences in your overall health, as issues will start to heal through autophagy.

Note: An interesting side effect many experience when their body is learning to switch to fat burning, is they can be cold often, even in the hot summer. Once your body adapts and can transition smoothly to fat burning mode, the cycles of cold dissipate.

A brief list of only SOME of things I have found relief from when my body could begin to really heal itself:

Chronic Migraines
Inflammation and swelling

Chronic Fatigue
Chronic Fasciitis
Tennis elbow
Back, neck and shoulder pain and aches
Crows Feet around my eyes
Disturbed sleep
Night sweats
PMS, bloating and cramping

I also want to touch on a few other things that may happen during the adjustment period that are common, just so you are aware. Some people report changes in sleeping pattern, either sleeping more or less, as their body adjusts to fasting and healing processes begin. This is usually resolved within a few weeks, with better and more sound sleep as the outcome. After becoming adapted, most people find they need less sleep than before, but it's more sound.

Some women report changes in their menstrual cycle in the beginning, but with many issues such as irregularity, PMS and severe cramping being finally resolved. See: www.idmprogram.com/women-and-

fasting-does-fasting-affect-your-cycle/.
Hair thinning can also happen in the case of sudden diet change or rapid weight loss. If this happens, you can either ride it out or slow down your weight loss. This can happen with any lifestyle change and is not specific to fasting. It will subside and hair will thicken again.

And just a little warning: MANY women with fertility issues have reported conceiving within just a few months of starting to fast. And many women have reported peri-menpause reversing as well. Some people report temporary issues like skin blemishes, and bouts of bowel irregularities as their bodies detox. If any problems persist or become painful or concerning, please see your doctor.

For a discussion on side effects see: www.idmprogram.com/fasting-basics-common-side-effects-of-fasting

There is one more important factor I want to stress for those who are looking to lose weight. Weight loss is never linear.

Fluctuations are a normal part of our weight management. I have had fluctuations as much as 4 pounds in a single day. So if you decide to track your weight, please keep a log and then average your weight over time. As long as you see an overall downward trend, then you are doing well. Don't let daily up and down fluctuations upset or disappoint you. Taking weekly measurements, seeing how clothes fit, and before and after pictures, gives a much more accurate picture of weight loss. For women in particular, they will likely lose inches before weight and many even gain in the first few weeks of IF, as their body adjusts. Please know, that it is also common to even gain a little weight in the beginning, as your body goes into protective mode and holds onto excess water. Don't let this concern you, as it will release once your body understands everything is ok.

Also keep in mind, these two things: weight that has been with you the longest, will be the hardest to get off. It's just that way, no matter what weight loss plan you try. So be patient. You didn't gain all the weight in a month, so don't expect it to come off in a month. Also, keep in mind that you may have insulin resistance and have to reset your weight set point. And this takes TIME. It's not an instant thing. But stick with it, because resetting your weight set point, is what will enable you to keep the weight off long term.

Sometimes for women in particular, especially those who've been carrying extra weight for a longer time, seem to respond better to another form of IF known as ADF. When there is insulin resistance, longer fasts, with longer eating windows, often work better to break the insulin resistance.

ADF

Another form of Intermittent Fasting is known as "Alternate Day Fasting" or ADF. This type of fasting has a different set of ratios: usually 5:2 or 4:3. The 5 stands for the number of days in a week that you eat, and the 2 is for the fasting days. The 4 is days eating, and the 3 is days fasting. People do this in different ways: but the most common approach would be an 8 hour window on their "up" days (eating days) and only have water, black coffee, black tea, green tea, on their "down" days (fasting days).

Some people will have one small meal under 500 calories on their "down" days, but many find this just makes them more hungry, and they do better to not eat at all on their "down" days. And if your goal is autophagy, then eating even a 500 calorie meal will halt it.

The main point of ADF is to have alternating days were the intake of food is widely different. And most people do not start with this type of schedule, but incorporate it after doing the daily fasting schedule for a while, so they can build up their fasting capability first. An example of a 4:3 ADF schedule might be:

Sunday, eat 2 meals within a 6-8 hour window.

Fast Monday all day

Tuesday eat 2 meals within a 6-8 hour window.

Wednesday fast all day

Thursday eat 2-3 meals within 6-8 hour window

Friday fast all day

Saturday eat 1-3 meals within a 4-8 hour window.

A 5:2 ADF schedule might look like:

Fast all day Monday

Eat 2 meals Tuesday within a 6-8 hour window

Eat 1 meal Wednesday within a 4 hour window

Eat 2 meals Thursday within a 6-8 hour window

Fast all day Friday

Eat 2 meals Saturday within a 6-8 hour window

Eat 2 meals Sunday within a 6-8 hour window

There are also ADF fasts that are 3x36, 3x42 and 2x48, which are 3 days of 36 or 42 hour fasts, and 2 days of 48 hour fasts, respectively. Or continuous ADF which is eating/fasting every other day. These should always be followed by a 6-8 hour, at least two meal eating window.

There are many different ways to do ADF, and it is highly customizable and it's only a matter of finding which works best for you. Because it encourages metabolic confusion, many people use ADF to break a plateau, increase weight loss or change things up. This is all personal choice and what works best for you. Dr. Fung encourages changing schedules up every so often, so that your body does not adapt. I myself have done everything from 16:8, to OAMD to ADF. If you remain on OMAD long term, you can run the risk of going into a calorie deficit and slowing your metabolism. So it is good to sometimes add in a TMAD (two meal a day) or 8 hour window, do a weekly 36-40 hr fast, or switch to ADF to ensure you are getting enough calories and nutrients.

Whichever type of fasting cycle you choose, I encourage you still change things up sometimes. If you follow a rigorous schedule, eating the same way at the same time every day, your body can eventually settle into it and cause a plateau. Keep some sort of metabolic confusion by switching things up every once in while. Have a longer window, change your window time, or throw in a longer fast. Just something to keep your body guessing.
See: www,ginstephens.com/all-blog-posts/can-your-body-adapt-to-your-fasting-plan

Recommended reads for IF are Delay, Don't Deny by Gin Stephens and Feast Without Fear, also by Gin Stephens. Delay, Don't Deny was the first thing I ever read about Intermittent Fasting, I recommend this book so much. It is a very easy read, and is not too "sciency". She is so relatable and this book is what got me on board in the first place.

Some recommended reads for ADF are The Every Other Day Diet by Dr. Krista Varady and The Alternate Day Diet by Dr. James Johnson. Delay, Don't Deny also has a good chapter on ADF.

Extended Fasting

There is a lot to be said for extended fasting. It is much more aggressive, and can be quite difficult for a lot of people. It is definitely not required, and it is usually recommended to be supervised by a doctor or nutritionist when doing anything beyond 72 hours. Though personally, I think that if you do not have major health concerns, most experienced fasters could easily do a 5-7 day ok on their own.

Benefits of a longer fast would be to burn through glycogen stores more quickly, and to promote increased autophagy, boosting healing. You will get there with Intermittent Fasting, it just takes longer, because you will burn through glycogen stores more slowly. So don't think this is something you have to do. But if you are confident in your fasting muscle, and have the will power, a longer fast can be highly beneficial. For seasoned fasters, a longer fast is a breeze. But if you aren't ready or still fairly new to fasting, it can be challenging.

Common longer fasts for IFers (Intermittent Fasters) are 36, 40 and 48 hours. Many will also eventually extend to 50, 56, 60, 65 and 72 hours. These types of fasts aren't really meant to be done frequently. If that is what you want, then it is better to just do the ADF style. However a single, weekly, biweekly (as in every two weeks), monthly, or quarterly longer fast can easily be incorporated. The benefit to these fasts, is to burn through glycogen stores more quickly, reduce insulin resistance, and to speed up the autophagy process for further healing.

Before doing ADF, I had used 24-48 hour fasts to boost my healing. I will tell you, early on, I started with several 24s, once a week for several weeks, and they went pretty well. Then I attempted a 48 hour. It didn't go so well. I had to stop at 41. I was ravenously hungry and was starting to not feel well. And honestly, I probably should have stopped at 36. So the next one, I decided I'd go with 36 because of my experience before, but ended up going to 40 hours because I was feeling pretty good. After that it got even easier. The next one after that was 46 and it was a breeze, and a 60 went smoothly.

So it gets easier once you've burned those glycogen stores up, and strengthened that fasting muscle. So don't feel bad or like you failed if you attempt a longer fast, and have to stop before your target time. Listen to your body. You'll get there. And keep in mind that refeeding is just as important as the fast. The general rule is that anything over 40 hrs, should be followed by a Tre of 6-8 hrs, for ½ the fasted time. So if you fasted for 4 days, you will need to eat 2 days of 6-8 hr windows, with two meals in each day.

I do need to mention some tips on breaking a longer fast. Anything 36-72 hours, break with something light and small. Like a greek yogurt, cottage cheese, avocado, tomato and cucumber slices, piece of fruit or bowl of soup or bone broth, then wait 30-60 minutes before diving into a meal. If I'm over 48 hours fasting, I may do this twice before having a meal. It's just something to let your stomach know to get ready to receive food again. This is to help prevent a lot of stomach problems frequently experienced when breaking a fast, such as stomachaches, bloating or diarrhea. It is not recommended to break a longer fast with eggs or nuts, though some people do without issue.

If you go over 72 hours and get into the range of fasting for multiple days, then you need to be even more cautious in breaking that fast. Usually starting with liquids such as watered down soup or bone broth. That is one reason why it is often recommended to be supervised for fasts over 72 hours. The longer your digestive system has been at rest, the more gently you need to wake it up again.

Dr. Fung uses extended fasting frequently in his clinic. His IDM Program offers counseling and coaching to help find the right and safest fast, especially for anyone with challenging conditions such as severe obesity, diabetes or fatty liver. You may notice Dr. Fung allows fasting aides or crutches for extended weight loss fasting beyond 3 days. These include homemade bone broth and pickle juice which are used for the immense electrolyte value during 5, 7 and 10 days fasts. Water only is protocol for autophagy fasting. You can find him on www.IDMprogram.com

There have been some fascinating studies on the affects of extended fasting and a great documentary on the subject is called "The Science of Fasting". They delve into MUCH longer fasts – 14, 21 and 40 days. Currently I do not plan on attempting these, but it doesn't take away from the science behind it. It is available on Amazon, and free to Prime members. It is really eye opening what the affects of fasts have on the body and brain for healing.

At this point, I want to encourage you watch an interview with Dr. Jason Fung. It wraps up everything talked about so far in a beautiful and understandable way. It is really worth the 1.5 hours. I had it saved for weeks before I "had the time" to sit and watch it. But if I had known what was in the interview, I would have made time immediately to watch it. You can find it on youtube by searching "Leptin & Insulin Resistance Balancing Tips W/ Jason Fung, MD. Or enter this link: https://youtu.be/jXXGxoNFag4.

Whether you plan an extended fast or not, I suggest watching a great series on youtube:
Life in the Fasting Lane 10 day fast with Eve Mayer. She chronicles her 10 day fast

each day and is guided and coached by Megan Romas of IDM Program along the way. It is full of valuable information.

A quick note on working out while fasting. It is perfectly fine to do, and actually even more beneficial, as while fasted, your body is making more HGH. However, if you are not yet fat adapted, working out while fasting can be difficult, since you will be running on glycogen stores. It is recommended to do light workouts during this adjustment period. After you have become fat adapted, working out will not only be much easier and more enjoyable, but performance will be enhanced by the burning of sustainable fat energy.
See: idmprogram.com/fasting-and-exercise-fasting-23/

Another great resource is a youtube video "All the Fasting Answers" with Megan Ramos. Https://youtu.be/-cAAzbqt95Y?list=LLDsfXn6qLHYfwq0bS-Hy4dA

Electrolyte Chart

Sodium	Headache, fatigue/weakness, dizziness, difficulty concentrating, nausea/vomiting	3000-7000mg 1 tsp salt=2335mg sodium. Use pure salt
Magnesium	Muscle cramps/twitching, irritability, insomnia, constipation	400mg citrate, glycinate, chloride or malate. remember not to use Oxide.
Potassium (remember it is not suggested to supplement potassium unless directed by a doctor or in the event of an extended fast beyond 72 hours).	Muscle cramps/weakness muscle twitching, heart palpitation, increased awareness of heartbeat rapid heartbeat, numbness/tingling	3000-4700mg citrate powder or bicarbonate capsule. Nusalt 1/6 tsp=530mg Cream of tartar 1 tsp=500mg 1/2avocado= 485mg

Listen to your Gut

Now that we've talked about when to eat, its time to talk about what to eat. I know some of you are thinking, "Please, I need you to tell me WHAT to eat!" and others are thinking, "Oh no, here it goes, now I'm going to be told what NOT eat". Well, I'm not going to do either. What I do want you to think about is, the opposite side of fasting, feasting!

I saw someone write once that they choose to call their lifestyle "Intermittent Eating" instead of Intermittent Fasting, because not only does it sound more palatable to the average person, but it's like the other side of the same coin. Some may find it hard to conceptualize the fasting part, but its much easier to wrap our brain around the eating part! Instead of concentrating on the I CAN'T eat for ____amount of time, think about I CAN eat for ____ amount of time!

Before continuing, I want you to stop reading and watch something. It will make what I am about to say so much clearer. It really will. There is a Tedx talk available on Youtube called "What is the Best Diet for Humans" by Eran Segal. You can search it or enter in the link: https://youtu.be/0z03xkwFbw4. I'll wait while you watch it.

Done? Great. This is why I am not going to tell you what to eat, or what not to eat. I do not know your body, your DNA, microbiomes or your diet history. But I am going to give you some of the keys I've learned into honing in on what YOU should be eating,

We've already talked about the CI/CO lie. If you want further study on this see:

www.scientificamerican.com/article/science-reveals-why-calorie-counts-are-all-wrong/ and go back to the links I proved earlier as well.

So we are not going to concern ourselves with how much or how many calories (or points, or carbs, or macros etc) we are eating in our window. From what we have learned about appetite correction, we know that will work itself out with time. And from the first chapter, we know that not every "diet" works for everyone. Some people have already found the foods that work well for them (which is why they want to push their eating style on you), but many haven't. And some even find that after starting to fast, they learn that foods they thought worked, actually don't, and vice versa. Many people find that food they thought they could or couldn't eat, including food sensitivities, change.

However, I will add here that there is ONE type of food that does NOT work for ANYONE. And that is chemically processed foods. As you saw in the video, chemically processed foods, actually change our microbiomes in our gut, leading to very negative effects. Now I know not everyone can always buy organic and cook from scratch or have access to a local farm to secure fresh foods from, but simple changes can make a big difference.

Start by reading labels, and compare the same product in different brands. Choose the one with the least amount of ingredients, and totally avoid ones with ingredients lists that are paragraphs long with words you can't even pronounce. Your body is not meant to process all of those chemicals and additives. They aren't even food, most of them are toxic, and they will alter your microbiome in a negative way. You want dinner rolls with your meal? Or a bowl of ice cream for dessert? By all means, have them! But just think about buying the ones with better ingredients. You Gut with thank you.

Note: Personally, as an added note, I also suggest staying away for corn syrup and high fructose corn syrup, as well as MSG, and watch out because they are in almost everything. As research has become abundant about the detrimental effects that HFCS and MSG has on our bodies, many companies are now leaving it out and even labeling their products as high fructose corn syrup free and MSG free. I encourage to seek out the research about this product and become informed. Also, artificial sweeteners, even the "natural ones" still spike your insulin, regardless if they are sugar free or zero calorie.

So when you begin to fast, I don't want you to worry about any type of "diet" to follow. Adapt to fasting first. Too much at once, can derail you and make you want to quit because it's just too hard. Baby steps. If you are accustomed to going through drive thrus, eating a lot of processed foods or having donuts for breakfast, then don't worry about that right now. Work on fasting first. Appetite correction has got your back. By the time you have achieved this, you will also have made progress on balancing your gut.

Our gut is a wonderful thing. As you fast, things will begin to adjust in your gut. You may go through a period of "cleaning out" when you spend quality time in the bathroom. If it becomes consistent, make sure you are hydrated adequately. If you are getting dehydrated during your fast, then jump into quick rehydrating when you eat, it can send you to the restroom. You may also have the opposite happen (if so, drink plenty of water and add some magnesium citrate to you window). I am a HUGE of fan probiotics. Many are available as supplements, but I prefer to get mine naturally through fermented food and drinks. This was a major step in my gut healing I mentioned about in the beginning.

And I still take care of my gut in this way everyday. If you aren't sure what foods are rich in probiotics, things like yogurt (with active cultures), sauerkraut, kimchi, miso, pickles and aged cheeses are great probiotic foods, and things like buttermilk, kefir and kombucha are great drinks. You can easily search online for a list. Try to add some kind of probiotic to your diet.

Along with appetite correction, as your gut heals, you will start to find your taste and reaction to various foods will likely change. When you used to crave those pop tarts, they suddenly don't seem that appetizing anymore. They definitely aren't worth opening your window for. You gain a new perspective on food. You become more in tune with flavors, smells and how you feel when you eat something. You begin to tell when something nourishes you or not. If you begin to experience things like stomachaches, fatigue, bloating, increased hunger or sugar cravings, or headaches after eating certain foods, you know that food item is not working for you.

Things can even taste different. You

notice you can't finish that huge plate of food, that you used to have no problem eating. You learn when to stop at satiety instead of going on until overly full. This usually happens naturally with fasting. If you would like to read a bit more about the difference between satiety and full see: https://alissarumsey.com/intuitive-eating/fullness-vs-satisfaction/.

Digging Deeper

For those who are already accustomed to fasting, or just are little crazy and want to address poor eating habits right off the bat, I'll talk about a couple of things. There is a fabulous way of eating, called Intuitive Eating. It's basically where you learn to listen to your body's signals when it tells you what kind of food to eat. This is actually pretty difficult to do if you haven't fasted, are insulin resistant, and your gut is all out of balance from dietary choices that don't work for you. As we saw in the Best Diet video, what we eat actually changes our microbiomes and you will continue to crave those things that are damaging to your body. So you really need to heal your gut and work on insulin resistance before this works. Fasting is a fantastic way to start. Once you've adapted to fasting, you'll notice your feelings towards food change. As you eat, pay close attention to how foods make you feel. What makes you feel energetic, light, peaceful and strong? Eat those foods. What makes you feel bloated, lethargic, cranky, or irritable? Don't eat those things. Which food fill you up satiety without that gross bloated feeling? And which foods leave you craving sugar or cause you to overindulge because they aren't satiating you? These are the clues into what works for you and what doesn't.

Concentrate on nutrient dense food, as they provide satiety for the body. Your body recognizes food by its nutrients, and gives you a clear signal when its full. It can not do that with processed food, which is why it's common to over eat it. Have you ever heard someone say, "wow I ate an apple and couldn't stop and I ate 40 apples"? Not likely, but we all know the situation of "I ate an oreo and couldn't stop and ate the whole pack". So be sure to include real, whole, nutrient dense food.

If your interested in going a step further, go ahead and start changing your eating habits. Like I said before, start with reducing processed foods and start reading labels. Even if you do nothing else, the difference this will make on your overall health will be tremendous.

If you want a starting place to take the next step (and many end up there naturally when they've fasted enough), is to adopt the Mediterranean way of eating. An interesting study was done on the people in the world who live the longest and are the healthiest. The top five places in the world are categorized into areas they called "The Blue Zones". There are two interesting things about these places: 1) they all eat extremely similar diets and 2) they are all foods that our good gut bacteria thrive on.

What are these foods? Do they count calories? Follow Ketogenic, Low fat, vegetarian or some type of special eating plan? Absolutely not. They eat, they enjoy, they celebrate, they don't stress about food. And their diets are rich in vitamins and minerals, very nutrient dense. All of them have fresh fruits and vegetables as the main portion of their meals. Imagine that, the natural food that God provided for us, is the most nutritious and life giving!.

They all also commonly eat some form of grains and carbohydrates, whether it be wheat, potatoes, sweet potatoes, rice, corn, beans, and/or legumes. These Blue Zones are spread over the world, so different varieties of these food group are available to them. They drink some alcohol almost daily (usually wine, but some places its other fermented drinks), and they consume water, coffee and tea on a daily basis. They usually have meat or fish several times a week and even have sweets and desserts several times a week. If you want to learn more about this fascinating study, visit www.bluezones.com. This can be a good starting point, if you want to change what your eating, and aren't sure where to begin. This is a great place to start and then tweak as necessary.

Another eating plan that many have had success with, is an elimination diet. The basis of these plans is to remove certain foods from your diet completely for a certain amount of time, and then add them back in slowly one by one and see how your body reacts. This is a great way to help pin point certain foods that you suspect might be giving you trouble, but aren't sure. If you have a food allergy, than it is obvious what you can't eat. But other foods may cause more subtle sensitivities, or cause an issue that you may not have related to food. Many people have been allergy tested and already know what they can't eat. But sensitivities can be different from allergies and not always picked up on. And like I said before, sensitivities and even allergies can change, when your microbiome changes.

I have not done one of these, so I can not provide you with much information on the best way to do it, or the best plan to follow. If you feel this is right for you, then I encourage you to go research it.

Currently I just follow Intuitive Eating. I have been fasting long enough, and I know my gut is balanced and healthy, so I pay close attention to how foods make me feel. Different signs can range from obvious to more subtle. If you get a bad stomach ache, or feel nauseated, or have excess gas, its pretty obvious something in that meal did not work for you. But I have had other reactions that aren't as in your face – corn syrup and high fructose corn syrup makes me feel jittery and my heart will pound. Many people feel this way with caffeine, but caffeine does not have this effect me.

This one took me time to figure out, because most people suggested it was "sugar" or "carbs". But I could have a dessert with unrefined cane sugar, raw sugar coconut sugar, honey, sucanat and even white sugar (though that one only in very small quantities) without that problem. I can eat breads and pastas made with organic unbleached whole grains, but not refined bleached white flour. I get bloated, cranky and crave sweet things. They key to intuitive eating, is paying attention to how you feel after eating and if you don't feel good and feel nourished, then something isn't working.

In this style, you will also be more in tune with what you are naturally craving. I'm not talking about the sugar or refined snack food cravings. Those are coming from a gut imbalance. I'm talking about real healthy food cravings. You can tell the difference between a healthy craving and an unhealthy craving by your body's response. If you eat what you are craving, and you are satiated and the craving stops, then you have fulfilled the nutrient your body needed. If it does not satiate hunger, and you continue to crave and thus overeat, it was an unhealthy craving. Some days, I will crave a huge salad full of veggies. Some days I will crave meat and potatoes. Sometimes I just want fruit, cheese, and nut plate and am fully satisfied. Other days I want a big three course meal, complete with a slice of cheesecake.

Some days I will eat one meal, other days I may eat two meals and other days I may not eat at all. I currently switch back and forth from OMAD schedule with my window varying anywhere from 1-5 hours to ADF. Several times a month, I may have a longer fast, followed by a nice long eating day. By the time you read this, I may be doing some other type of schedule. After becoming fat adapted and achieving appetite correction, I can trust my body to tell me not only what to eat, but how much to eat and when. No worries about calories, or carbs, or points or grams. I eat! I love eating in my window, and I fully enjoy and savor every wonderful, delicious thing I eat! And if its not wonderful and delicious, its just not worth eating.

I hope you will find that freedom too.

IMPORATNT NOTE:
I will add that Dr. Fung recommends HFLC (high fat, low carb with protein being 20-30%) way of eating for obesity, sugar addiction, insulin resistance, fatty liver, diabetes and many other of his patients. For severe obesity, insulin resistance, diabetes etc. Dr Fung believes it crucial to begin with a combination of HFLC and fasting. If this is you, please read more about that in his books *The Obesity Code* and *The Diabetes Code* and in his blog idmprogram.com. Please also look into his counseling and coaching services and be sure to work with your doctor.

Post Script

Supplements, Medications, and OTC's

Vitamins and supplements should be reserved to your window. MTC oils, collagen, bulletproof coffee, protein or dietary shakes, drink powders and things like lemon wedges, herbs and essential oils ingested should all be saved for your window. Items in the grey zone can be tried after a period of clean fasting for at least 4-6 weeks. You can however apply essential oils, creams, salves etc. topically while fasting.

Ibuprofen is never recommended on an empty stomach, but acetaminophen and paracetamol are regarded as safe for an empty stomach. If you have questions or concerns about this, ask your doctor or pharmacist.

All prescription medications should be taken as directed by your doctor. If you have a prescription that is required to be taken outside of your eating window, and you can not adjust your window to accommodate it, many people recommend taking the medication with a small amount of a high fat, unsweetened food like plain greek yogurt, plain cottage cheese, or mashed avocado. It does break your fast, but at least it will have an extremely low glucose response, causing your insulin spike to be not as high as with other foods. If you have questions or concerns about this, ask your doctor or pharmacist.

Precautions

It is not recommend to fast if you are pregnant or breastfeeding.

It not recommended that anyone under 18 fasts. If you have concerns about an overweight child, a few simple and safe changes can be made.

*Keep eating within a 12 -13 hour period (no bedtime snacks)
*Reduce or eliminate highly processed foods, junks foods and foods with refined sugar. Also cut out sugary drinks such as sodas and juice drinks.
*Cut out snacking, especially of things like chips and cookies. A child beyond toddler years can do well on a a good solid and nutritious 3 meals a day.

Anyone with a history of eating disorders, should never embark on any eating or diet regimen without support and close supervision from their doctor.

If you have major health concerns or diseases, please work with your doctor before attempting any kind of fasting. Dr. Fung and other doctors and nutritionists, use fasting to reverse many metabolic disorders including type 2 diabetes, heart disease, fatty liver disease, thyroid disorders, insulin resistance, high blood pressure, PCOS and more. Those on these plans, are generally supervised so blood work can be checked regularly and medication can be adjusted as necessary.

If you are medication dependent, please talk to your doctor before starting this, or any other diet or eating program. If your doctor does not support fasting in any way - I'm not talking about if they support fasting, but you have restrictions based on your personal profile, - then I suggest you seek out a doctor that supports fasting, to supervise you on your journey. If your doctor or someone in your life that is one, may be open to learning about fasting, I suggest you refer them to Dr Jason Fung's website www.idmprogram.com and his books: The Obesity Code, The Diabetes Code, and The Complete Guide to Fasting.

IDMProgram.com also offers coaching for those with complications and concersn and would like more in depth guided fasting.

The Rest of Your Body

Another step I recommend taking, is to also look at the ingredients in your household products. Check your cleaning supplies, detergents, cleansers and hygiene products. It very easy to simply purchase the product with the least amount of indecipherable ingredients, just like with your food. And it doesn't have to be more expensive either. As the market is growing for non toxic household and personal supplies, they have become more affordable and to easy to access. There are even recipes online to make your own at extremely low costs. Any thing that comes into contact with your skin, or ingested in your mouth, deserves a closer look to see exactly what it in them.

Recommended Reading and Other Resources

Delay, Don't Deny by Gin Stephens. This is a very easy, casual read and a great place for beginners or those first starting to learn.

Feast Without Fear by Gin Stephens. Another easy and casual read, that delves into the food we eat in addition to fasting.

The Obesity Code by Jason Fung, MD. This is much more of a technical read, and is chock full of scientific information. This is great for those who really want a deeper medical understanding, and perfect for anyone with a medical background, who wants to know the science behind insulin and fasting.

The Complete Guide Fasting by Jason Fung, MD. A more in depth look at the power of fasting, explanations and directions for fasting protocols, and troubleshooting.

The Diabetes Code by Jason Fung, MD. A must read if you or someone you love has diabetes and wants to reverse it naturally.

The Clever Gut Diet by Michale Mosley. Learn about your gut and how it relates to your overall health.

The Power of Appetite Correction by Dr. Bert Herring. Learn more about appetite correction and the power it has to change your health.

<u>Websites</u>: check out their blogs and articles.
www.Ginstephens.com
www.idmprogram.com
www.dietdoctor.com

<u>Podcasts</u>: Great listening with a wealth of information.

"Intermittent Fasting Stories" Gin Stephens
"The Intermittent Fasting Podcast" Melanie Avalon
"The Obesity Code Podcast" Dr. Jason Fung and Megan Ramos

<u>Support Groups: Facebook</u>:
These groups are excellent sources for support while on your fasting journey. They all have an array of files to read that answer many questions, as well as posts for support and answering questions and troubleshooting. I highly recommend them. I belong to them all!

*Delay, Don't Deny: Intermittent Fasting Support
*Delay, Don't Deny: Advanced Book Support Group
*One Meal A Day IF Lifestyle
*The Obesity Code Network: Fasting Support with Megan Ramos and Dr. Jason Fung
*The Dr. Jason Fung Fan Club – Fasting Support

Some great reference books for healing with natural herbs and plants:
Nutritional Herbology by Mark Pederson
Intergrated Guide to Essentail Oils and Aromatherapy

Additional resources:
Health Related Mindsets by Kathie Walters -great book about how sometimes health problems can be linked to mindsets.
Life Sea Minerals, sea mineral supplement – I love using this as electrolyte support.
Glow: All Natural and organic face and skin oils (handmade by me!)
These are available at:
www.kathiewaltersministry.com

www.ingramcontent.com/pod-product-compliance
Lightning Source LLC
Chambersburg PA
CBHW050554280326
41933CB00011B/1842